Notebook JOURNAL

THIS BOOK BELONGS TO

____

IF FOUND PLEASE CALL

____

Owthorne Notebooks

www.ingramcontent.com/pod-product-compliance
Lightning Source LLC
Chambersburg PA
CBHW072203280526
45788CB00002B/862
* 9 7 8 1 0 8 7 4 0 1 2 8 7 *